HONEY AND OIL:

Essential Uses and benefits of honey and oil

Charles Friddle

TABLE OF CONTENT

CHAPTER 1

Honey and Raw honey
Honey is a thick, sweet syrup made by honey bees.
It's loaded with healthy plant compounds and has been linked to several health benefits.

Raw Honey has been used as a remedy throughout history and has a variety of health benefits and medical uses. It's even used in some hospitals as a treatment for wounds. Many of these health benefits are specific to raw, or unpasteurized, honey.

Most of the honey you find in grocery stores is pasteurized. The high heat kills unwanted yeast, can improve the color and texture, removes any crystallization, and extends the shelf life. However, many of the beneficial nutrients are also destroyed in the process.

If you're interested in trying raw honey, you might consider buying it from a trusted local producer.

CHAPTER 2

Types of Honey

While all honey comes from bees, not all honey is the same. Where bees source their nectar affects the taste, sweetness level, and color.Differentiate between different types of honey, such as manuka, organic, and raw honey, and learn some helpful tips on how to keep your honey looking and tasting its
best!

According to the National Honey Board, there are over 300 different varieties of honey
produced worldwide. All honey has a sweet taste, but there are several key factors that make
each type of honey unique, such as color and flavor profile.

Below, we'll break down 10 of the most popular types of honey and their distinct flavors.

1. Clover Honey

Saturated with the aromatic, mild flavor of clover blossoms, clover honey is the best-known honey variety with the largest annual production. Grown in Canada, the United States, Sweden, and New Zealand, this popular honey has a sweet, mild taste with a hint of cinnamon and a light golden color. Although clover honey doesn't contain as many antioxidants as darker varieties (such as buckwheat and manuka), it's the perfect all-purpose honey to keep on hand in your establishment for all your tableside needs.

Recommended for table use, cooking, and baking

Commonly used in desserts, sauces, meats, sweet bread, yogurt, and cereal

2. Wildflower Honey
Wildflower honey features a select blend of wild blossoms and flowers. Because wildflower honey is collected from any variety of wildflowers depending on the season and region that they're in bloom, it may originate from any country that grows honey.
Its taste varies depending on the flowers it is created from. However, it's typically slightly darker than other honey varieties, adding a robust flavor to baking recipes.
Recommended for cooking and baking
Commonly used in muffins, meats, and loaves of bread

3. Acacia Honey
Acacia honey is created with the nectar from black locust trees, also known as false acacia trees. For this reason, it is sometimes sold as "locust honey" in the United States. The honey features a sweet, delicate flavor with a hint of vanilla and a light, almost transparent color.
Likely due to its higher fructose content, acacia honey takes longer to crystallize. As a result, acacia honey is a great choice for smaller establishments that may take a long time to finish a jar of honey.
Recommended for table use, cooking, and baking
Commonly used in yogurt, cereal, teas, drinks, and desserts

4. Alfalfa Honey
Largely produced in the United States and Canada, the alfalfa honey variety is created with nectar from bright purple alfalfa blossoms. The final product is a light, herbal-flavored honey with delicate, mildly sweet undertones.
Alfalfa's smooth texture and mild taste are akin to clover honey. Because Alfalfa is slightly less sweet, however, it is more ideally used for cooking applications. Add it to pastries and loaves of bread as a healthy alternative to sugar.

Recommended for table use, cooking, and baking
Commonly used in teas, dressings, and sauces

5. Buckwheat Honey
Dark and bold, buckwheat honey is collected fresh from the small white blossoms of the buckwheat grain. It's grown in the United States, France, Canada, Japan, and the Netherlands.
Typically compared to blackstrap molasses, this honey variety is characterized by an earthy aroma and a rich amber color. It has a stronger and heartier taste than lighter honey varieties, and it's also higher in antioxidants. Because of its bold flavors, buckwheat honey is best used for baking and cooking. Products baked with this golden honey will dry out less quickly and be less likely to crack than those baked with traditional sugar.
Recommended for cooking and baking
Commonly used in honeycakes, loaves of bread, and sauces

6. Creamed Honey
While it's not technically a type of honey, creamed honey denotes a special way of preparing honey. Also known as spun honey, it is made by storing honey at a temperature of around 55 degrees Fahrenheit and letting it crystallize. Creamed honey has a richer, creamier texture than traditional honey. It also typically has a much lighter color than liquid honey from the same flower. The crystals in creamed honey create a smooth and easily spreadable product. It's a great addition to breakfast spread offerings and adds interest to any menu.
Recommended for table use, cooking, and baking
Commonly used as a spread on bagels, toast, and biscuits

7. Manuka Honey

Manuka honey is produced in Australia and New Zealand by bees that pollinate the native Manuka bush. This honey offers a mildly sweet taste with a subtle nutty flavor. A slightly bitter aftertaste offsets the initial sweetness. While most honey has natural antibacterial qualities, manuka honey has greater amounts of antibacterial ingredients than most other types of honey. This Australian honey protects against damage from bacteria, boosts the production of special cells that repair damaged tissue, and eases pain and inflammation.
Recommended for table use, cooking, and baking
Commonly used as a spread on toast, bagels, and biscuits, as well as in yogurt and cereal

8. Eucalyptus Honey
Gathered from the flowering eucalyptus trees of Australia, this distinctive honey has a sweet flavor offset by cool undertones of fresh eucalyptus.
Eucalyptus honey has a slightly medicinal scent. Because of its menthol-like properties, this honey is great for soothing coughs, colds, and upper-respiratory infections. Eucalyptus honey features mild.
Recommended for table use, cooking, and baking
Commonly used on toast and in teas and pastries

9. Orange Blossom Honey
Fresh from the spring blossoms of Florida's orange groves, orange blossom honey features light citrus undertones. It has a golden color and a wholesome, sweet taste and aroma.
The citrusy elements of orange blossom honey add an exciting element to baking endeavors. Try blending it with softened butter, orange rind, and lemon rind to create orange blossom honey butter, which is sure to become a popular menu item.
Baker's special honey is drizzled onto a pastry.
Recommended for table use, cooking, and baking
Commonly used in drinks and on biscuits, pancakes, and pastries

10. Baker's Special Honey
Baker's special honey is a blend of classic honey varieties. Featuring a deep amber color and rich flavor, this honey has a more robust taste than lighter, tableside honey.
As its name implies, baker's special honey is the perfect alternative to standard sugar in baking recipes. This honey variety is also used for brewing batches of mead, a trendy fermented beverage made from yeast and honey.
Recommended for cooking and baking
Commonly used in whole wheat bread, pastries, and BBQsauces.

What is Honeycomb?
Bees create honeycombs to house their larvae, honey, and pollen. The hexagonal cells that
makeup honeycomb is made of beeswax and contains honey in its purest, rawest form.
Can You Eat Honeycomb?
Yes! In fact, people have been eating honeycomb for thousands of years. Not only is honeycomb a tasty,all-natural snack, but it is also rich in vitamins and minerals.

How to Eat Honeycomb
The raw honey and waxy cells of the honeycomb are both edible. Much like honey, honeycomb varies in taste depending on the types of nectar the bees gathered.
Honeycomb is delicious and eaten on its own. Or, try eating honeycomb in a variety of other unique ways, including:
Thinly slicing it on toast
Using it to top salads
Using it to garnish cocktails
Adding it to a charcuterie board

Expert Tip
Honey is a charcuterie board essential. Consider pairing your honey or honeycomb with aged
cheeses featuring nutty undertones such as Parmigiano-Reggiano and sharp cheddar. Honey
also pairs well with tangy, acidic cheeses like feta and goat cheese, as it subdues these bold flavors.

How Long Does Honey Last?
Honey can last forever if properly stored in a sealed container and kept away from moisture. Moisture will contaminate the honey and cause it to spoil, giving it a sour taste. As long as it's kept at room temperature, however, it will be safe from harm. As a result, you may use your honey long after its "best by" date has passed.

Honey Crystallization
As time goes by, you may notice that your honey has lost its liquid consistency and formed small crystals. This is perfectly normal! In fact, it's common for honey to crystallize over time.
Wooden honey dipper in a glass jar of crystallized honey

Why Does Honey Crystallize?
Because honey is made of water and a mix of sugars (mainly glucose and fructose), the sugar can precipitate out of the honey over time. As this happens, the water separates from the sugar, creating the appearance of small crystals.
To prevent honey from crystallizing, store it in an airtight container in a cool, dry location. It's also best to avoid refrigerating honey, as this speeds up the process of crystallization.
Is Crystallized Honey Safe to Eat?
Honey can still be consumed in its crystallized form. Some people even find that crystallized honey has a richer flavor and is easier to spread.
Jar of honey in crystallized form with a honey dipper

How to Decrystallize Honey

Learn how to soften honey with these two easy methods.

1. Boil water in a

 2. Place your closed container of honey in a large glass container and pour the hot water over

   the container.

3. Let the container of honey soak for several minutes, or until it has softened and liquified.

4. Use more hot water if the honey has not softened after several minutes.

Another method is to soften honey in the microwave.

1. Place honey in a microwave-safe container.

2. Microwave over medium power for 30 seconds at a time, stirring each time.

3. Repeat until the honey is fully softened.

CHAPTER 3

The essential use of honey for health

Health benefits of honey and raw honey.
Here are some health benefits raw honey has to offer:
1. A good source of antioxidants
Raw honey contains an array of plant chemicals that act as antioxidants. Some types of honey have as many antioxidants as fruits and vegetables. Antioxidants help to protect your body from cell damage due to free radicals.

Free radicals contribute to the aging process and may also contribute to the development of chronic diseases such as cancer and heart disease. Research showsTrusted Source that antioxidant compounds in raw honey called polyphenols have anti-inflammatory effects that could be beneficial in protecting against a number of conditions associated with oxidative stress.

The raw version of honey can also contain bee pollen and bee propolis, which may have added benefits. A 2017 review of studiesTrusted Source suggested that raw honey may have potential protective effects for the respiratory, gastrointestinal, cardiovascular, and nervous systems, and even has potential in cancer treatment.

2. Raw honey nutrition
Raw honey's nutrition content varies by its origin and other factors. Generally, one tablespoon or 21 grams of raw honey contains trusted Source 64 calories and 17 grams of sugar. Raw honey also contains trusted Source smaller amounts of the following micronutrients (or, vitamins and minerals):

calcium

magnesium

manganese

niacin

pantothenic acid

phosphorous

potassium

riboflavin

zinc

In addition, raw honey is a source of varying amounts of amino acids, enzymes, and other beneficial compounds.

3. Antibacterial and antifungal properties
ResearchTrusted Source has shown that the propolis in raw honey has antifungal and antibacterial properties Trusted Source.

The potential for both internal and topical treatments using raw honey is significant. Honey's effectiveness as an antibacterial or antifungal varies depending on the honey, but some varieties are being studied for specific therapeutic uses such as against Candida-associated infections

4. Heals wounds
A 2018 review of studies found that honey has antimicrobial properties. A 2017 review of studiesTrusted Sources also suggested that honey, propolis, and royal jelly may have potential health benefits for microbial inhibition and wound healing.

Keep in mind that the honey used in research settings is medical grade, meaning it's inspected and sterile. It's not a good idea to treat cuts with honey you buy from a store. Always speak with your doctor before using honey for any medical purposes.

5. Phytonutrient powerhouse

Phytonutrients are compounds found in plants that help protect the plant from harm. For example, some keep insects away or shield the plant from ultraviolet radiation.

The phytonutrients in honey are responsible trustee Sources for its antioxidant properties, as well as its antibacterial and antifungal power. They're also thought to be the reason raw honey has shown immune-boosting and anticancer benefits. Heavy processing in regular honey can destroy these valuable nutrients.

6. Help with digestive issues
Honey is sometimes used to treat digestive issues such as diarrhea, though research to show that it works is limited. It may have potential as a treatment for Helicobacter pylori (H. pylori) bacteria, though, a common cause of stomach ulcers.

It also contains beneficial prebiotics, meaning it nourishes the good bacteria that live in the intestines, which are crucial not only for digestion but overall health.

7. Soothe a sore throat and cough
Honey is an old sore throat remedy that soothes the ache and can help with coughs. Add it to hot tea with lemon when a cold virus hits.

Though more research is needed, a 2021 review of studiesTrusted Sources suggested that honey could be superior to other forms of care for the improvement of upper respiratory tract infections.

A 2016 study also suggested that the antibacterial and anti-inflammatory properties are effective in helping a sore throat.

8. Brain benefits

There may even be some cognitive benefits to raw honey. The polyphenols in honey may be able to counterTrusted Source inflammation in the hippocampus, the part of the brain involved in memory.

The antioxidant and anti-inflammatory effects can benefit many parts of the body, including brain health.

Are there any risks?
In addition to beneficial prebiotics and nutrients, raw honey can also carry harmful bacteria such as Clostridium botulinum. This is particularly dangerous for babies. The Centers for Disease Control and Prevention (CDC)Trusted Source advises that honey should never be given to an infant younger than a year old.

Symptoms of botulism poisoning in infants may include:

constipation
slow breathing
sagging eyelids
absence of gagging
loss of head control
paralysis that spreads downward
poor feeding
lethargy
weak cry
In adults, symptoms can include an initial short period of diarrhea and vomiting, followed by constipation and more severe symptoms, such as blurred vision and muscle weakness. Speak with a doctor if you experience any of these symptoms after eating raw honey.

You'll also want to avoid honey if you have an allergy to honey or bee pollen.

How to choose the right raw honey
You'll want to look for honey that says "raw" on the label or comes from a farm that can verify that it hasn't been pasteurized. Honey comes in many varieties with labels like "natural," "organic," and "pure," but none of those indicate that it's raw.

Look for a label that says "raw" specifically and look out for any added ingredients like artificial sweeteners. Mainstream and organic grocery stores, health food stores, and farmer's markets are all places to look for raw honey.

How do I store raw honey?
Honey doesn't expire very easily but it can become contaminated in certain circumstances. Store honey in a tightly sealed container away from light and extreme temperatures.

After a while, your honey may start to crystallize. This is completely safe but can make it look grainy and sugary. You can warm it just slightly to melt the crystals, but know that higher temperatures can cook the honey, removing its raw properties and causing it to darken in color.

If your honey has changed color drastically or smells off, throw it out.

Raw honey is best described as honey "as it exists in the beehive".

It is made by extracting honey from the honeycombs of the hive and pouring it over a mesh or nylon cloth to separate the honey from impurities like beeswax and dead bees.

Once strained, raw honey is bottled and ready to be enjoyed.

On the other hand, the production of regular honey involves several more steps before it is bottled — such as pasteurization and filtration.

Pasteurization is a process that destroys the yeast found in honey by applying high heat. This helps extend the shelf life and makes it smoother.

Also, filtration further removes impurities like debris and air bubbles so that the honey stays as a clear liquid for longer. This is aesthetically appealing to many consumers.

Some commercial honey is additionally processed by undergoing ultrafiltration. This process further refines it to make it more transparent and smooth, but it can also remove beneficial nutrients like pollen, enzymes, and antioxidants.

Moreover, some manufacturers may add sugar or sweeteners to honey to reduce costs.

CHAPTER 4

Essential uses of honey for Beauty

Honey long ago claimed the throne as the queen bee of the beauty world. Skeptical? Just take a trip to Sephora or the drugstore for proof of the multiple beauty uses of honey. You'll see it in face masks, shampoos, lotions, lip balms, and more.
Why, exactly though, is honey used in so many beauty products? "Honey has natural healing properties," says Mona Gohara, MD, associate clinical professor at Yale Department of Dermatology, particularly for wound healing. It can also promote collagen-building, Dr. Gohara adds, making it a great anti-ager.

That's not all the sweet stuff can do: "Honey has natural antiseptic, antibacterial, and anti-inflammatory properties," says Dendy Engelman, MD, a New York City-based dermatologic surgeon.
Still, that doesn't mean the stuff that comes in the bear-shaped bottle at the grocery store is going to magically fix all your skin problems. Carly Stein, the founder of Beekeeper's Naturals, says the best honey for beauty use is raw and unpasteurized.

Stein recommends sticking with buckwheat honey (a dark honey made from the nectar of...well, buckwheat) because of its high antioxidant levels. And if you're having trouble finding some, Stein says to just look for a dark, raw honey—the darker the honey, the higher the antioxidant count and better for your beauty routine.

Ways Honey Can Up Your Beauty Game.

Curious about how honey can help you step up your beauty game? Look no further:

1. Moisturizing Face Mask

"With its moisturizing and soothing effects, raw honey can hydrate the skin, leaving it soft, radiant, and glowing," says Ildi Pekar, celebrity facialist and owner of Ildi Pekar Skin Care. "The sugars in honey act as natural humectants and emollients that increase the water content and reduce dryness in the skin even after they have been washed off and (for all the label-readers out there), if you can find raw honey with a high concentration of other bee products such as royal jelly, which is prime for boosting collagen; propolis, which is anti-inflammatory and antibacterial (so, a major win for acne-prone skin); or pollen which "contains a compound called rutin that helps drain the capillaries" and smooths out blemishes, you can take your routine up a notch.

Try it: Apply raw honey directly on the skin and leave it on for up to 20 minutes, then rinse and massage it off thoroughly with water.

2. Gentle Exfoliant

Since raw honey crystalizes over time, the tiny granules act as a gentle exfoliant. They start to break down when they come into contact with water and the heat of your skin making for a gentler scrub than that of the harsher store-bought stuff. And since it's antibacterial, you can use it for your daily face wash.

Try it: Warm the honey in your hands by rubbing it between your fingers first, then apply it directly on the skin in circular motions. Leave it on for a few minutes before massaging it off with a wet towel.

3. Scar Fader

Finger, Hand, Line, Yellow, Thumb, Gesture, Personal protective equipment, Clip art,

.

The antioxidant properties in honey (particularly buckwheat honey) nourish damaged skin, helping the scar healing process, according to Stein. And for the added bonus of anti-inflammation, keep an eye out for honey infused with propolis—it can help tone down the look of stretch marks and skin discoloration.

Try it: Massage raw honey directly to the affected area in a circular motion for one to two minutes, then rinse it off.

4. Wound Healer
Honey's natural antiseptic properties help prevent infections and protect wounds, says Dr. Engelman, which can reduce scarring and cut down on healing time. The antioxidants in honey (particularly Manuka honey) are more than ready to serve as a natural remedy to nourish your damaged skin and bring it back to its unblemished glory.

Try it: Apply raw honey directly to the affected area and let it sit for one to two minutes, then rinse it off. If that's a little too sticky, hit up the drugstore for a branded honey-infused wound treatment which won't be as thick.

5. Acne Spot Treatment
Buckwheat honey is a great DIY remedy for acne. It's an anti-inflammatory, which helps reduce the redness and swelling of pimples, says Stein, and its antibacterial properties can help fight acne-causing bacteria especially if it's infused with propolis. "Also, because honey keeps the skin well-hydrated and balanced, it helps control the production of oil," adds Pekar.
Try it: Apply raw honey directly on the breakout and then rinse it off after 10 to 15 minutes

6. Bath Soak

Up your relaxation goals and take a honey-infused soak. Honey's hydrating powers will leave skin silky soft, says Pekar.

Try it: Make it at home by mixing two big tablespoons of raw honey into one cup of hot water until the honey is dissolved. Pour it into a tub of warm water to soak. You can also use a pre-made version if that's more of your style.

7. Cuticle Moisturizer
Since honey is a natural humectant (aka it draws moisture into the skin), it can help keep the skin around your cuticles happy and peel-free.

Grab a bottle of honey that's packing royal jelly, another bee product, Stein says, since it's a collagen-builder. That added ingredient will bring new life to your nails and strengthen the skin around them.

Try it: Rub raw honey over each cuticle and leave it on for five to 10 minutes before rinsing it off.

8. Everyday Conditioner
"Honey is naturally a perfect conditioner because it's a humectant and retains and attracts moisture, keeping your hair feeling smooth and healthy," says Felix Fischer, celebrity hair artist. "Your strands will feel soft, and nourished, and have plenty of life and bounce."

Try it: Mix one-quarter cup of organic raw honey with just enough fresh water to thin it out so you can spread it around your hair. Work it into damp hair after you shampoo for a few minutes, then rinse with warm water.

9. Lip Balm

Lip, Red, Face, Mouth, Facial expression, Nose, Cheek, Smile, Clip art, Eye.

Everything that makes honey a great skin moisturizer makes it great for chapped lips, too. "The hydrating benefits mixed with natural enzymes, antioxidants, and minerals work well to moisturize lips," Pekar says.

Try it: Apply raw honey directly to lips, leave on for a few minutes, then wash off.

10. Hydrating Hair Treatment

Honey can prevent your hair from drying out because it is very effective in retaining moisture and keeping locks soft and bouncy. It acts as a natural softener, says Fischer

Try it: Make a banana and honey hair mask by combining two very ripe bananas, half a cup of unprocessed honey, and one-quarter cup of olive oil. Blend the ingredients until smooth then apply this to your hair and scalp. Leave it on for about 20 to 25 minutes, then rinse the mask out with cool or lukewarm water and shampoo. Comb through the hair to get rid of any remaining mask and rinse again. This mask can be used two to three times a month.

11. Sleep Aid

"When you eat honey it causes a slow, steady spike of insulin," Stein explains, which converts to serotonin and melatonin, two chemicals that help you fall asleep. And, if you're one to wake up in the middle of the night, a tablespoon of honey will help you stay asleep since "[honey] helps to stock the glycogen in the liver—" something the brain needs to keep you asleep for a dreamy eight hours.

Try it: Eat a spoonful of honey 15 minutes before bed. Or, if waking up in the middle of the night is causing trouble, have a spoonful then.

12. Burn Relief

The anti-inflammatory, antibacterial, and moisture-restoring properties of honey are super soothing on an irritated and irritating burn (even a sunburn). Plus, its thickness acts as a barrier from any infections that might try to make their way into the burn, so no need to cover it with gauze after you apply the honey.

Try it: Clean the burn, then rub a few drops of honey onto the area and let sit for as long as you like (which—warning—will get messy) before rinsing off. Reapply as needed.

CHAPTER 5

Essential uses of honey sexually

Benefits of Honey for Sexuality:
 Honey
Honey is a magical substance made by bees from the nectar of flowers and is a symbol of
procreation. You might have heard about the medicinal properties of honey but did you
know that honey is also good for sexuality? The most potent honey is from bees that gather
nectar from aphrodisiac flowers like marjoram, orchids, or jasmine. An example of potent
honey that you can try if you want to gain honey benefits for sexuality is Honey, made
from the nectar of Sidr trees.

The use of honey as an aphrodisiac actually dates back to ancient times. It has been
associated with love and sex in ancient books like the Bible and Kamasutra. Even the word
honeymoon came into existence because of its ability to stimulate sexual desire and
prowess. Is honey beneficial for men? yes, most newlyweds would be given a drink made
from honey and milk that would boost potency in men because the honey benefits for
sexuality are so widely known.

Honey benefits for sexuality
Drinking Honey is beneficial for your body in a variety of ways as it improves digestion

as well as increases bone and muscle mass. Honey is also rich in
antioxidants which
reduces the risk of cancer, strokes, and heart attack. There are various
good chemicals
present in honey like Boron, Vitamin B, Nitric oxide, natural sugars,
and several others
which help increase stamina, boost testosterone levels, and give you a
boost of
energy in a short period of time. It also helps in increasing sexual
desire and sexual

Honey for Stamina
Honey is said to restore energy, enhance physical stamina and lessen
the risk of
cardiovascular diseases. Consuming as little as 85 grams of honey for
stamina every day
significantly boosts the level of nitric oxide in the blood, which is the
chemical responsible
for penile erections. That's why homeopaths recommend ginger and
honey in case of
erectile dysfunction. Nitric oxide also helps in maintaining glucose
levels, glycogen
restoration, and increasing blood flow, leading to a boost in stamina
while working out
or during coitus. Start consuming milk and honey for stamina daily
and you will see the
difference in your stamina and sexual prowess in a short time. Honey,
is also known as an
aphrodisiac, so it increases sperm count, and also it has been regarded
as a natural fertility
booster for generations.

Boost your Testosterone Levels with Honey

Honey is also a prominent source of Vitamin B and Boron. These nutrients are responsible

for a strong skeletal structure and better muscle coordination. But that's not all, Boron is

also responsible for the usage of testosterone, estrogen and Vitamin D. Honey for men is a

boon in disguise as it is rich in a chemical known as chrysin that blocks the conversion of

testosterone into estrogen and ultimately boosts the testosterone level in your body. A Healthy drink made from honey for men

One of the best ways to gain all the honey benefits for sexuality is by consuming honey in

the following ways:

• Honey and Warm Water

A glass of honey and warm water boosts metabolism and keeps body fat under control.

Having this mixture first thing in the morning will give you a boost of energy that will help

you wake up even better than a cup of coffee.

• Honey and Milk

Milk is a rich source of Calcium, Vitamin D, and Proteins while Honey is a rich source of

Vitamin B, Boron, and antioxidants. So, it makes complete sense to mix them and create a

sweet drink that will give you enough vitamins and minerals to keep your body fit and

healthy.

• Honey Tea

Tea is known for its soothing properties and healthy antioxidants, honey is also known for

these properties as well. So combining them both gives a boost to the medicinal

properties as well as relaxes your body.

- Honey Lemonade

After a long workout or a tiring day at work, a honey lemonade drink will help you treat
sore muscles and give you a boost of energy meanwhile maintaining the level of body fats and increasing the level of good hormones in your body.
After knowing so many honey benefits for sexuality, you must be planning on getting tons
of honey for your kitchen. But you should not start gulping down bottles of honey at a time
as it will not only increase your blood sugar level but also lead to weight gain. It is
necessary to have honey in moderation with the rest of your diet to increase your sexual
prowess and for a stamina boost.

CHAPTER 6

Oil

Cooking oil is a plant, animal, or synthetic fat used in frying, baking, and other types of cooking. It is also used in food preparation and flavoring not involving heat, such as salad dressings and bread dips, and in this sense might be more accurately termed edible oil. Cooking oil is typically a liquid at room temperature, although some oils that contain saturated fat, such as coconut oil, palm oil, and palm kernel oil are solid. There is a wide variety of cooking oils from plant sources such as olive oil, palm oil, soybean oil, canola oil (rapeseed oil), corn oil, peanut oil, and other vegetable oils, as well as animal-based oils like butter and lard. Oil can be flavored with aromatic foodstuffs such as herbs, chilies, or garlic.

Oils are the basis for many favorite recipes and play a major part in various cooking techniques, from sautéing and frying to roasting and baking.

While many recipes specify which oil to use, some don't. And believe it or not, you may actually get a superior meal by experimenting with something other than what's called for.

CHAPTER 7

Essential Uses of oil for health

Here's an overview of the health benefits and best uses of common cooking oils.

Oils: Health benefits, smoke points, best uses, and how to store properly

1. Extra-virgin olive oil
Quite possibly the most well-known and frequently used cooking oil, extra-virgin olive oil, or EVOO, has earned its reputation as a healthy, versatile fat. It makes an excellent choice for its antioxidant content, heart-healthy fats, and its links to cancer prevention.

Because of these benefits, and its widespread availability, you may find yourself using EVOO for absolutely every type of food prep.

But its low smoke point (the temperature at which it begins to degrade and release damaging free radicals) means it's not always the best oil to use for cooking — at least not cooking at temperatures above 375°F (191°C).

For this reason, EVOO is often recommended for colder dishes like dips, salads, and dressings.

Store in an opaque container in a cool, dark place.!

2. Light olive oil

Extra-virgin may get the most attention in the world of olive oils, but its "light" cousin contains many of the same health-boosting properties.

Light olive oil has a far higher smoke point of about 470°F (243°C). Therefore, it's ideal for high-temperature cooking, like sautéing, roasting, and grilling.

Light olive oil can also be used in baking, but be aware that its flavor may be overpowering. And don't be fooled by its name. This olive oil doesn't contain fewer calories than other varieties. Rather, "light" refers to its more neutral taste.

Store in an opaque container in a cool, dark place.

3. Coconut oil
Like most other oils, coconut comes in two varieties: refined or unrefined (also known as "virgin").

Refined coconut oil has a smoke point of 450°F (232°C). It works well for sautéing or roasting and has a neutral, light-coconut taste.

Virgin coconut oil, on the other hand, offers a more signature coconut flavor and can be used at temperatures up to 350°F (177°C). Both are also suitable for baking with a 1:1 ratio of butter or other oils.

Coconut oil has seen its share of controversy over its healthiness recently, so check out our analysis of the evidence around its health benefits.

Store in a glass container in a cool, dark place.

4. Canola and other vegetable oils
Now a kitchen staple, canola oil was developed in the 1970s by researchers at the University of Manitoba — hence the prefix "can" for Canada.

While other vegetable oils come from a blend of vegetables (which, depending on labeling, may remain a mystery), canola oil is always derived from rapeseed plants.

The refining process of both canola and other vegetable oils leaves them with a neutral taste and medium-high smoke point of 400°F (204°C). This makes them useful for stir-frying, sautéing, grilling, frying, and baking.

Health information about canola and other vegetable oils can be conflicting, so check out our guide to their benefits and drawbacks.

Store in a cool, dark place.

5. Avocado oil
If you know that avocados are chock-full of healthy monounsaturated fats, you won't be surprised to learn that their oil is, too.

In addition to a high content of these good fats, avocado oil boasts the highest known smoke point of any plant oil — 520°F (271°C) for refined and up to 480°F (249°C) for unrefined. It's a rock star for frying, searing, roasting, and grilling.

Though avocado oil is considered a carrier oil that lets other flavors shine, choose the refined version if you prefer a mild, unobtrusive taste.

Store in a cool, dark place or in the refrigerator for longer preservation.

6. Peanut oil
There's a reason peanut oil is so often used in Thai, Chinese, and other Asian cuisines. The refined variety, with a smoke point of 450°F (232°C), is wonderfully conducive to high-temperature stir-frying.

It also works well in large-batch frying, which is why the food industry heavily relies upon it for menu items like french fries and fried chicken.

Unrefined peanut oil, on the other hand, has a smoke point of 320°F (160°C). Add it to dressings or marinades for extra flavor. See our guide for information on peanut oil's health effects.

Store in a cool, dark place.

7. Sesame oil
Sesame oil just may be the unsung hero your cooking needs. With plenty of monounsaturated fats and antioxidants, it rivals olive oil as a healthy choice for cooking.

A mid-range smoke point of anywhere from 350 to 400°F (177 to 204°C) means it can be used in stir-frying and sautéing as well as adding flavor as a condiment.

Store in the refrigerator for best results.

CHAPTER 8

Vegetable oil and seed oil
Are Vegetable and Seed Oils Bad for Your Health?

The consumption of vegetable oils has increased dramatically in the past century.

Most mainstream health professionals consider them healthy, but vegetable oils may cause health problems.

Their health effects vary depending on what fatty acids they contain, what plants they are extracted from, and how they are processed.

This article looks at the evidence to determine if vegetable and seed oils are bad for your health.

What are they and how are they made?
Edible oils extracted from plants are commonly known as vegetable oils.

In addition to their use in cooking and baking, they're found in processed foods, including salad dressings, margarine, mayonnaise, and cookies.

Common vegetable oils include soybean oil, sunflower oil, olive oil, and coconut oil.

Refined vegetable oils were not available until the 20th century when the technology to extract them became available.

These are extracted from plants using either a chemical solvent or an oil mill. Then they are often purified, refined, and sometimes chemically altered.

Health-conscious consumers prefer oils that are made by crushing or pressing plants or seeds, rather than those produced using chemicals.

Consumption has increased drastically
In the past century, the consumption of vegetable oils has increased at the expense of other fats like butter.

They are often labeled "heart-healthy" and recommended as an alternative to sources of saturated fat, such as butter, lard, and tallow.

The reason vegetable oils are considered heart-healthy is that studies consistently link polyunsaturated fat to a reduced risk of heart problems, compared with saturated fat.

Despite their potential health benefits, some scientists are worried about how much of these oils people are consuming.

These concerns mostly apply to oils that contain a lot of omega-6 fats, as explained below

You may want to avoid vegetable oils high in omega-6
It's important to note that not all plant oils are bad for your health. For example, coconut oil and olive oil are both excellent choices.

Consider avoiding the following plant oils due to their high omega-6 contents:

soybean oil
corn oil

cottonseed oil
sunflower oil
peanut oil
sesame oil
rice bran oil
Both omega-6 and omega-3 fatty acids are essential fatty acids, meaning that you need some of them in your diet because your body can't produce them.

Throughout evolution, humans got omega-3 and omega-6 in a certain ratio. While this ratio differed between populations, it's estimated to have been about 1:1.

However, in the past century or so, this ratio in the Western diet has shifted dramatically and may be as high as 20:1.

Scientists have hypothesized that too much omega-6 relative to omega-3 may contribute to chronic inflammation.

Chronic inflammation is an underlying factor in some of the most common Western diseases, such as heart disease, cancer, diabetes, and arthritis.

Observational studies have also associated a high intake of omega-6 fat with an increased risk of obesity, heart disease, arthritis, and inflammatory bowel disease.

However, these associations don't necessarily imply a causal relationship.

Studies investigating the effects of omega-6 fat consumption generally do not support the idea that these fats increase inflammation.

For instance, eating a lot of linoleic acids, which are the most common omega-6 fat, doesn't appear to affect blood levels of inflammatory markers.

Scientists do not fully understand what effects omega-6 fats have on the body, and more studies are needed.

However, if you are concerned, avoid oils or margarine that contain oils high in omega-6 fats. Olive oil is a good example of a healthy cooking oil that's low in omega-6.

They are sometimes high in trans fats
Commercial vegetable oils may also contain trans fats, which form when the oils are hydrogenated.

Food producers use hydrogenation to harden vegetable oils, making them solid like butter at room temperature.

For this reason, vegetable oils found in margarine are commonly hydrogenated and full of trans fats. However, trans-fat-free margarine is becoming increasingly popular.

However, non-hydrogenated vegetable oils may also contain some trans fats. One source looked at vegetable oils in the United States and discovered that their trans-fat contents varied between 0.56% and 4.2%.

A high intake of trans fats is associated with all sorts of chronic diseases, including heart disease, obesity, cancer, and diabetes.

If a product lists hydrogenated oil as an ingredient, it likely contains trans fats. For optimal health, avoid these products.

Vegetable oils and heart disease
Health professionals often recommend vegetable oils for those at risk of heart disease.

The reason is that vegetable oils are generally low in saturated fat and high in polyunsaturated fat.

The benefits of reduced saturated fat intake are controversial.

However, studies show that replacing saturated fat with polyunsaturated fat reduces the risk of heart problems by 17%, but it has no significant effects on the risk of death from heart disease.

Furthermore, omega-3 polyunsaturated fatty acids appear to have a greater benefit than omega-6.

Nutritionists have raised concerns about the high amounts of omega-6 found in some vegetable oils. However, there is currently no solid evidence showing that omega-6 fats affect your risk of heart disease.

In conclusion, a moderate intake of vegetable oils seems to be a safe bet if you wish to reduce your risk of heart disease. Olive oil may be one of your best options.

Vegetable oils generally seem to be healthy sources of fat.

Hydrogenated vegetable oils that are high in unhealthy trans fats are an exception to this.

Some nutritionists are also concerned about the high amounts of polyunsaturated omega-6 fats found in certain vegetable oils.

Olive oil is an excellent example of a healthy vegetable oil that's low in omega-6. It might be one of your best options.